EAT FIT

A Nutritional Blueprint For Healthy Living

Toluse Francis

ACKNOWLEDGEMENT

To everyone who has played one role or the other in my journey towards this project, I say THANK YOU!

DEDICATION

To everyone who seeks knowledge to nutrition and healthy eating do I dedicate this book.

FORWARD

I consider this book a gift to whomever reads it. Many books on the subject are grandiloquent, this is not one of them.

It is simple to read, easy to understand, it is short, yet fully loaded with information.

I recommend this book to anyone who wants a head start on how to eat, what to eat and why to eat.

Toluse put in a lot of effort into making this book a reality, I commend him and I also congratulate everyone who will have the opportunity to read it.

Remi Owadokun
Certified Health Coach
Amazon Best Seller of 'How I lost 40kg'

Their Experience...

When I got a copy of Toluse's book Eat Fit... I didn't know what to expect. But by chapter 3 I was hooked. Toluse brings an interesting perspective to the conversation about health and wellness. I find the premise that I can basically improve the quality of my life by simply paying close attention to what I eat was ground breaking for me. I highly recommend Eat Fit as required reading for anyone interested in improving the quality of their life and the results they produce in the market place

Victor Ekpo Bassey,
Founder Highly Paid Experts Network

This book is jammed packed full of useful information on eating healthy. I really like how it is simply and easy to follow. Toluse has managed to uncomplicate a topic in an area which is becoming quickly too complicated by too much choice and "new fad diets" hitting the market each day. This book is a must read to clear out the myths, the non-sense and get back to basics.

Kimberly Manning -
Mindset and Health Coach Australia

Written in simple, clear grammar and held up in less than 60 pages, this book will show you in clear, non-jargonical terms how to stay fit via the things that enter into your mouth.

Look, as entrepreneurs you and I know the greatest vehicles we have to take us to the great future we are building is a sound mind and a healthy body. If our health breaks down, all those talks about raising capital, about securing market shares, about conquering the world, building wealth, or about disrupting the market will just be a pie in the sky. I recommend this book to every entrepreneur

Chinonso Ogbogu-
Founder, The SM Group and Converner
#TheIncubatorsPRO

Toluse Francis is passionate about helping people make better health decisions. In a world of ever increasing, and ever more confusing, choices, this book offers much-needed guidance. Read it!

Doc Ayomide,
Mind Health Specialist

Table of Contents

INTRODUCTION

Few die of hunger, many die of eating.
- Benjamin Franklin

When people hear the word diet, they quickly think weight loss. This is probably due to usage of the word by those who have themselves misunderstood it or never understood it in the first place.

Healthy eating means consuming the right quantities of foods from all food groups to lead a healthy life. The meals we eat, play a great role in our lives. They determine how we look, how we feel and sometimes how we behave.

Look at this:

A developing child has no right over what he/she eats, and so it is till a child reaches a certain age. Probably until they become teenagers, which means until they get to that age range of 13 - 19 years old, they remain at the mercy of whatever they are given. The sad part is that, if they are fed wrongly for that period, they would have had the wrong diet for thirteen (13) years. Isn't that huge?

So let's do some maths here.
Let N represent number of years
Let T represent number of times you eat per day
With this, imagine you eat just twice a day for thirteen years (remember my previous analogy) multiplied by number of times you eat.

Thus,
Unhealthy Eating = N*T =13*2 = 26

Perhaps that's outrageous, right?

Let us half the number of years to say out of 13 years, only 6 years of terrible or unhealthy eating. This amounts to 12.

What this means is that for 13 years, you have dealt a heavy blow on your organs and every tissue of your body.

Can this be prevented? Yes but the choice is up to you.

We have the power over what we eat. Our decision is based on different factors such as climate, what you do, age to mention just a few.

Nutritional needs differ, and attention must be paid to this if we intend to keep body and soul together.

This book aims to open the eyes of its beholder to the importance of healthy eating. The world as a whole must realise that all our body needs to function and work well is dependent on healthy eating. We need to eat with a purpose rather than eat because we have to eat.

Eating habits also need to be looked at hence the reason for its highlight in this book. You would also gain knowledge into few recipes based on age, work type and stage of life, e.g., pregnant women.

It has been written with a global view hence no biased statement or impracticable meal suggestions therein.

As you flip through the pages of this book, keep a clear mind and be open to learning and practice as well

Thanks for reading

Toluse Francis
Founder, Eat Fit Academy
© 2016

Chapter One

EAT RIGHT, Eat Healthy

Change means that what was before wasn't perfect.
People want things to be better.
— Esther Dyson

Food is a necessity of every living creature and as such, it is important that we eat right.

Eating right is the key to living healthy.

A few examples:

Eat foods high in unsaturated fats: Saturated and trans fats (I'll explain what these mean later) will help you gain weight, but they'll also increase your cholesterol and your risk of heart disease. Unsaturated fats, however, contribute to reducing your risk of heart disease and boost your immune system. Make sure every meal you have includes some fat.

Eat whole wheat or grain carbohydrates. Carbohydrates act as energy sources for the body. If you don't burn off the energy, it will be stored as fat and help you gain weight. After fat, carbs are important contributors to weight gain, so you'll need plenty of these in your diet.

Replace white products with whole wheat bread, pasta, and brown rice. Include carbohydrates in all your meals to help in your weight gain as well as prevent constipation.

Use full-fat dairy products: Dairy is essential for your diet because it has calcium and vitamins. Most dairy products come in reduced-fat varieties, but you'll want the full-fat versions to increase your calorie and fat intake. Drink whole milk and eat cheese and yogurt made from whole milk.

Cook with butter instead of oil to give yourself another boost of fats. Enhance foods with calorie-rich ingredients. You can continue eating many of the foods you normally do but make them help your weight gain by adding a few ingredients. Some healthy and efficient options include:

Add hard-boiled eggs to salads.

Add cheese to sandwiches, eggs, and salads.

Eating Resolutions

To experience the needed change in our lives, we must change.

This will often include changes in what, how and when we eat. I will share with you, resolutions to help you change how you eat.

Eat more vegetables: vegetables are good for the body as they possess nourishing vitamins and help prevent indigestion.

Eat less fats: fats have nutritive value and contribute to growth and development, but they are bad in excess.

Do more home-made meals and less dining out.

Avoid mindless eating. Eat when you are hungry and don't multi-task.

Take that snack far from sight. Take healthy meal breaks when at work. If you must snack, do it only when famished and not out of boredom.

Eat smart at restaurants. Don't let yourself be too hungry before eating so you don't overeat. You could share with a friend.

Eat less sugar. Replace sugary drinks with unsweetened tea or water.

Try to eat breakfast every day. No matter how little.

Plan to eat right.

Be moderate at parties. Don't stay too close to foods serving points. Eat before going to reduce temptation.

Keep track of what you eat to help measure if you have kept to your goal

Learn to say NO. This is part of the discipline you have to deal with to eat healthily.

Plate size matters: you eat less with smaller plates.

Don't rush food. Eat slowly so your brain can tell you when you are full.

Support helps. Ask a friend, coach, or family member to join you. They can hold you accountable.

Make one healthy goal at a time and reward yourself when you succeed.

Chapter Two

Food Needs and Body Changes

Those who have no time for healthy eating will sooner or later find time for illness.
- Edward Stanley

You don't need a silver fork to eat good food.
- Paul Prudhomme

Food is simply sunlight in cold storage. John Harvey Kellogs

Age plays a role in healthy eating decisions. What you ate as a child, for instance, may not be eaten as an adult. Adults over 50 can feel better immediately and stay healthy for the future by choosing healthy foods. A balanced diet and physical activity contribute to a higher quality of life and enhanced independence as you age.

As you age, your food needs change. Growth and development, wear and tear of body tissues, changes in your mental activity account for these amendments.

Your body food needs as you grow.

Fruit – Whole fruits beat juices for fibre and vitamins. Aim for 2 portions or more each day. And instead of apples and bananas, every time, go for colour-rich pickings like carrots or melons.

Colourful Fruits are Attractive

Veggies – Colour is your friend here: dark, leafy greens (kale, spinach, broccoli) and orange or yellow vegetables (carrots, squash, and yams) are antioxidant-rich.

Calcium – Adequate calcium intake prevents osteoporosis and bone fractures. Older adults can get their recommended calcium requirement from milk, yogurt, or cheese, or non-dairy sources like tofu, broccoli and almonds, oranges, etc.

Grains – Be smart with your carbs: whole grains offer more nutrients and fibre than processed white flour. If you're not sure, look for pasta e.g., spaghetti, bread, and cereals that list "whole" in the ingredient list.

Protein – Adults without kidney disease or diabetes need 1 to 1.5 grams per kilogram of bodyweight. Divide protein intake equally across meals. And vary your protein sources instead of relying on red meat: including more fish, beans, peas, eggs, nuts, seeds, and low-fat milk and cheese.

Water – As we age, dehydration is likelier: our bodies don't regulate fluid as well, and the sense of thirst is less sharp. You can post a note in your kitchen to remind you to sip water every hour and with meals. This helps avoid urinary tract infections and constipation.

Vitamin B – After 50, the stomach produces less gastric acid, making it difficult to absorb the vitamin B-12 you need to for blood and nerve vitality. Consider fortified foods or a vitamin supplement for your recommended daily intake (2.4 mg).

Vitamin D – Sun exposure and certain foods (fatty fish, egg yolk, and fortified milk) provide most of our vitamin D— essential for absorbing calcium and boosting muscles. With age, our skin synthesizes vitamin D less efficiently, so consult your doctor about supplementing your diet with fortified foods or a multivitamin, especially if you're very large or get little sun.

Chapter Three

Digestion

Digestion is simply taking the good and leaving the rest..
- Toluse Francis.

Bad digestion is the root of all evil. - Hippocrates.
I am convinced that digestion is a great secret of life..
- Toluse Francis

You need more fibre as you age.

Eating foods high in dietary fibre can do so much more than keep your regular exercise. It can lower your risk of heart disease, stroke, and diabetes, improve your skin, help you lose weight, and boost your immune system and overall health. With age, though, digestion becomes less efficient, so it's important to include enough fibre in your diet. After age 50, women should aim for at least 21 grams of fibre per day, men at least 30 grams a day. Unfortunately, many don't get even half those amounts.

A few tips:

In general, the more natural and unprocessed the food, the higher it is in fibre.

Good fibre sources: whole grains, wheat cereals, barley, oatmeal, beans, nuts, vegetables (carrots, celery, and tomatoes), and fruits (apples, berries, citrus fruits, and pears)—further reason to add more fruit and vegetables to your diet.

An easy way to add more fibre: start your day with a high-fibre content meal like whole grain cereal. Just switching your breakfast cereal from corn flakes to bran can add about 6 extra grams. If you're not a fan of high-fibre cereals, try adding a couple of tablespoons of unprocessed wheat bran and fresh or dried fruit to your favourite cereal.

Whole fruits beat fruit juice for fibre and fewer calories. For instance, a 25 cl glass of orange juice (like the small juice packs) contains about 110 calories and almost no fibre, while one medium fresh orange contains about 3g of fibre and only 60 calories. Peeling can reduce the amount of fibre in fruit, so try to eat the peel of apples and pears.

Liven up dull salads with nuts, seeds, kidney beans, peas, or black beans. You can also make tasty high-fibre additions to soups and stews by adding peas, beans, lentils, and rice.

Tips for Healthy Eating

You need to get into the habit of eating healthy. It's gradual, though, not something you start all of a sudden.

Reduce salt to increase water output and reduce high blood pressure. Look for the "low sodium" label, and season meals with garlic, herbs, and spices instead of salt.

Take "good fats." Reap the rewards of olive oil, avocados, salmon, walnuts, flaxseed, and other monounsaturated fats which protect your body against heart disease by controlling "bad" LDL cholesterol levels and raising "good" HDL cholesterol levels.

Avoid "bad" carbs. Bad carbohydrates—also known as simple or unhealthy carbs—are foods such as white flour, refined sugar, and white rice that have been stripped of all bran, fibre, and nutrients. They digest quickly and cause spikes in blood sugar levels leading to short-lived energy. For long-lasting energy and stable sugar levels, choose "good" or complex carbs such as whole grains, beans, fruits, and vegetables.

Look for hidden sugar. Added sugar is often hidden in foods such as bread, canned soups and vegetables, pasta sauce, instant mashed potatoes, frozen dinners, fast food, and ketchup. Check food labels for forms of sugar: corn syrup, molasses, brown rice syrup, cane juice, fructose, sucrose, dextrose, or maltose. Opt for fresh or frozen vegetables instead of canned goods, and choose low-carb or sugar-free versions of products such as bread, pasta, and ice cream. Try to avoid artificial sweeteners as well—it's healthier to sweeten drinks with honey, or use whole fruit or fruit juice to sweeten dishes.

Cook smart. Preserve nutrients in veggies by steaming or sautéing (frying at relatively high heat) in olive oil. Forget boiling—it drains nutrients.

Think Japanese. Take a tip from Japanese food culture and try to include five colors on your plate. Fruits and veggies rich in colour correspond to rich nutrients (think: blackberries, melons, yams, spinach, tomatoes, zucchini). This attractiveness of colour is what makes the Japanese foods inviting.

Chapter Four

Meal Plans for Different Types of Work

Enjoy the fruit of your labour.It is health that is real wealth.
- Mahatma Gandhi

Office Workers

Gaining weight when you are at a desk for endless hours is easy.

Losing it is not.

We were born to move! Yes, just breathing or shifting a computer mouse around burns calories, but not enough to compensate for the number we consume every day. Sad, maybe, but true.

Studies reveal that desk-bound jobs are amongst the worst for packing on the pounds, no matter how dedicated we may be to lowering calorie content in our meals and snacks. The nutritional content of the meals and snacks matter more than the number of calories.

To keep your metabolism firing while you are sedentary, you need a diet with more fats than you are probably used to consuming and a whole lot less starchy carbohydrates.

Here are your diet secrets:
- Limit Starch. Carbohydrates should always feature in a healthy meal or snack, but starchy types (bread, pasta, rice and other grains) must be carefully monitored as they upset blood sugar levels, prompting weight gain when we are sedentary for many hours. Get the bulk of your carbohydrates from vegetables and limit starch to one or two meals or snacks per day.
- Plan Ahead. This obviously depends on how predictable your day is, but a lunchbox filled with delicious and nourishing goodies not only beats fast food sandwich and crisps hands down but also keeps hunger at bay for hours and reduces the chance of a mid-afternoon energy dip.
- Avoid Cravings. It's all too easy to reach for a sugary snack when you are at the desk and need a little something to keep you focused and energised for a while, but the resulting blood sugar surge merely encourages a greater need for more all too soon.
- Make your snacks protein-rich. Also, consider a supplement to blunt cravings.

Labour Intensive Workers

The strength and energy levels of anyone who performs hard physical work on a regular basis is directly affected by what they eat. Meal plans become just as important as punctuality to work. A healthy, smart, all-inclusive meal plan can add new verve to a workday.

Here are your diet secrets:

•   Good Carbohydrates. When your body needs energy for work, it turns to calories. During intense physical labour, as much as 85 percent of those calories can come from carbohydrates. Foods that contain bad carbs, like potatoes or sugar (energy and carbonated drinks), offer a short boost of energy, that is followed by a hard crash and a run-down feeling. Good carbs can be found in brown rice, whole grain pasta and beans, and will keep you energized for hours.

•   Good Proteins. Intense strain on muscles tears the fibres within them. The body responds by sending healing cells to the tear site, ultimately becoming one with them. With the addition of these new cells, muscles grow back larger and stronger. This process is driven by protein, and without a steady influx of fresh protein throughout the day, muscles remain stagnant in size and strength. The United States Department of Agriculture recommends that regularly exercising adults eat 0.6 g protein daily for every kilogram of bodyweight. Healthy foods like salmon, grass-fed beef and chicken can keep fat levels down and protein up.

• Caloric intake. The USDA also recommends that men ages 19 to 50, who exercise each day vigorously, eat 3,000 calories per day to maintain healthy energy levels. Just two meals daily, 1,500 calories each, will slow metabolism significantly, resulting in bouts of low energy between meals. It is better to spread calories out throughout the day to ensure a steady influx of calories, or fuel: consider three square meals daily, with small healthy snacks between meals, for consistent energy levels.

• Timing. To get your body ready and energized before work, eat a substantial, well-rounded breakfast a few hours ahead, to enable the body to absorb all necessary nutrients. Working too soon after large meal forces the body to reserve energy for digesting the food while you are working, putting you at an energy disadvantage.

Healthy Eating For Different Stages

Ideal diets change with different life stages. This ranges from pregnant to lactating mothers.

Pregnant Women

A foetus takes in what the mother takes, so this is of particular importance.

A pregnant woman could take a little snack as breakfast and a substantial meal for supper during the first trimester, to ease morning sickness while a large morning quantity and small night serving in the final trimester help with heartburn. Since no safe limit has been established for alcohol, abstinence is a woman's best bet.

Weight is also an important thing to take note of during pregnancy. If a woman does not gain enough weight, her baby won't either, placing the new-born at high risk for health problems. Optimal weight gains of 11.3kg to 13kg in a slender woman helps ensure a healthy-sized baby. Underweight women should gain more weight, or approximately 12kg to 18kg.

Overweight women should not attempt to use pregnancy as a way to use up extra body fat since stored body fat is not the stuff from which babies are made. A modest weight gain (7kg to 11kg) is recommended for these women. Weight gain should ideally increase from very little in the first trimester to as much as a 0.5kg a week in the last two months of pregnancy.

Diet Secrets

Eggs.

Eggs contain lots of proteins plus over 12 vitamins and minerals. They are also rich in choline, which promotes your baby's overall growth and brain health. Eggs are cheap and versatile.

Beans.

You already know the importance of protein in pregnancy, but you may not yet value fibre as a new best friend. Pregnancy slows your gastrointestinal tract, putting you at risk for constipation and haemorrhoids. Beans are not only protein- and fibre-rich, it's also rich in iron, folate, calcium, and zinc.

Sweet Potatoes.
Sweet potatoes get their orange colour from carotenoids; plant pigments that our bodies convert to vitamin A. Sweet potatoes are also an excellent source of vitamin C, folate, and fibre. And like beans, they're inexpensive and versatile.

Popcorn as Whole Grains.
Popcorn is a whole grain. Whole grains are important in pregnancy because they're high in fibre and nutrients, including vitamin E, selenium, and phytonutrients (plant compounds that protect cells).

Calcium.
Calcium should be a regular part of meals in pregnancy because babies need it to form and develop of bones and healthy skin. Yoghurts are an excellent source, and also, help keep your bones healthy, thereby providing for babies' needs without sacrificing your health.

Dark green, leafy vegetables.
Note, leafy vegetables, like spinach, in particular, not just vegetables.
They are loaded with vitamins (including A, C, and K), and nutrients like the all-important folate. They also promote eye health.

Rainbow diet. Green, red, orange, yellow, purple, and white.
Try lots of colours in your fruits and vegetables so you and your baby get a variety of nutrients.

Red.

Tomatoes, cranberries, raspberries, pomegranates or beets: all are packed with antioxidants such as vitamins A (beta-carotene) and C, manganese and fibre, making them great for your heart and overall health. Red apples also have Quercetin (/'kwɜrsɪtɪn/ is a flavonol found in many fruits, vegetables, leaves and grains. It can be used as an ingredient in supplements, beverages, or foods), which seems to fight colds, flu, and allergies. Also, tomatoes, watermelon, and red grapefruit are loaded with lycopene, said to be helpful against cancer.

Orange.

Citrus fruits are loaded with the antioxidant vitamin C and carrots with vitamin A (beta-carotene) for improved eyesight. They also contain potassium, fibre and vitamin B6 for general health.

Yellow.

Bananas include manganese, potassium, vitamin A, fibre and magnesium.

Chapter Five

SUGAR

Eat less sugar, you are sweet enough already
-Toluse Francis

Sugar is the generalized name for the sweet, short-chain, soluble carbohydrates common in food. They are carbohydrates (carbon, hydrogen, and oxygen) and come from different sources. Simple sugars (monosaccharide) include glucose (aka dextrose), fructose and galactose. Table or granulated sugar is sucrose, a disaccharide, which breaks down in the body into fructose and glucose. Other disaccharides are maltose and lactose. Sugars with longer chains are called oligosaccharides. Chemically different substances, like sweeteners, may have a sweet taste, but are not classified as sugars.

Most plant tissues contain sugars but are only present in enough concentration for extraction in sugarcane and sugar beets.

Lots of foods have higher sugar contents than many of us realise. Here are a few of these seemingly delicious foods.

Fat-Free Salad

Fat-free salad dressings are often laden with sugar: that's how manufacturers can ensure flavour after eliminating the fat. So they end up with calories from sugars like honey and concentrated fruit juice. There's sometimes as much as 8 grams of sugar (2 teaspoons) per 2 tablespoons of dressing. I recommend ditching fat-free dressings altogether and going with dressing in canola or olive oil as the top ingredient and (like tomato sauce) very little added sugar or none at all. These fat-containing dressings have more calories but are worth it because canola and olive oils are heart-healthy fats that help lower LDL cholesterol (the "bad" cholesterol). Use all dressings in moderation, though, because their calories add up quickly.

Smoothies

Smoothies are thick beverages made from blended raw fruits, are very popular now, and they might seem like a great way to add fruit and dairy to your diet. Most commercially prepared smoothies, however, have added sugars lurking in them.

One major brand boasts 38 grams of sugar (9½ teaspoons) and 230 calories in a single-serving bottle! Granted, some of these sugars come from the naturally occurring lactose in low-fat milk and fructose from blueberry juice, but sugar is also the second ingredient listed after milk. Smoothies help with fat prevention and are highly recommended in weight loss therapies.

Rice

Rice is one of the most consumed food today worldwide, and it has a high level of sugar. Foods with a high glycaemic (sugar) index like rice are more likely to leave you unsatisfied after your meal. A 2002 article in the American Journal of Clinical Nutrition shows that significant amounts on a regular basis make you hungrier and crave more foods, eventually leading to overweight and obesity. Keep a food diary and note how hungry you feel after eating different meals to help you catch this connection.

Carbonated Drinks

Carbonated Drinks are rich in sugar amongst other things. It is the sugar content that keeps bringing you back to take that Coca-Cola or Fanta.

As a quick reminder, carbonated drinks are so called because they have carbonated water

$H_2O(l) + CO_2(g) = CO_3(aq)$

Water + Carbon Dioxide = Carbonated Water

It is this carbonated water that gives the gaseous feel to the drinks which give the 'pop' sound when you uncork the bottle or container.

Even the alcohol consumed isn't free from sugar neither are the fruit juices; the only difference is that the sugars in the juices are naturally occurring from the fruits.

Chapter Six

Cholesterol and Foods
That Lower It

Change means that what was before wasn't perfect. People
want things to be beer.
— Esther Dyson

What if I told you cholesterol isn't all bad?

Cholesterol is a waxy substance that comes from two sources:
your body and food. Your body, and especially your liver,
makes all the cholesterol you need and circulates it through
the blood. But cholesterol is also found in foods from animal
sources, such as meat, poultry and full-fat dairy products.
Your liver produces more cholesterol when you eat a diet high
in saturated and trans fats.

Excess cholesterol can form plaque between layers of artery walls, making it harder for your heart to circulate blood. Plaque can break open and cause blood clots. If a clot blocks an artery that feeds the brain, it causes a stroke. If it blocks an artery that feeds the heart, it causes a heart attack.

There is Good and Bad Cholesterol.

Bad cholesterol: LDL cholesterol is considered "bad" because it contributes to plaque, a thick, hard deposit that can clog arteries and make them less flexible, a condition known as atherosclerosis. If a clot forms and blocks a narrowed artery, heart attack or stroke can result.

Peripheral artery disease can develop when plaque build-up narrows an artery supplying blood to the legs.

Good Cholesterol: HDL cholesterol is considered "good" because it helps remove LDL cholesterol from the arteries. Experts believe it acts as a scavenger, carrying LDL from the arteries and back to the liver, where it is broken down by passing out of the body. Up to one-third of blood cholesterol is carried by HDL. A healthy level of HDL cholesterol may also protect against heart attack and stroke while low levels of HDL cholesterol have been shown to increase the risk of heart disease.

Here are foods that can help lower cholesterol.

Chocolate: Dark chocolate contains flavonoids, antioxidants that help lower LDL levels. Just be sure to eat in moderation, as chocolate is also high in saturated fats and sugar. Cooking with dark, unsweetened cocoa powder offers similar heart-healthy effects.

Avocados: These provide oleic acid, which helps lower bad cholesterol. Try putting a few slices on a turkey sandwich, or adding them to a salad. Avocado oil, which has a subtle, sweet flavor, can also be used in place of other oils. You can ask your fruit vendor for one.

Red Wine: Red wine contains resveratrol (found in red grape skin), which may prevent damage to blood vessels by reducing the risk of blood clots and lowering LDL. Too much alcohol can cause a host of other health issues, however; so while a glass of red wine at dinner is fine, don't overdo it.

Tea: Black and green teas contain potent antioxidants that may reduce cholesterol levels. Green tea typically contains more of these antioxidant powerhouses, as it is made from unfermented leaves and is less processed. Just go easy on the cream and sugar.

Nuts: Nuts are high in polyunsaturated fatty acids, so almonds, walnuts, or pistachios can help reduce LDL levels. Try sprinkling them on salad, or as a snack. Just be sure to choose the low-salt option, and not more than 1.5 kg a day -- nuts are also high in calories. For almonds, that's about 30, or 1/3 cup.

Wholesome Whole Grains: Barley, oatmeal and brown rice have lots of soluble fibre, which helps lower LDL cholesterol by reducing cholesterol absorption. Try switching out your regular pasta for the whole-grain version, or use brown rice instead of white. Top your morning oatmeal with high-fibre fruit, like bananas or apples, for an added cholesterol-busting kick.

Go Fishing: Fish like salmon and sardines are rich in omega-3 fatty acids, which reduce triglycerides in the blood. Aim for 0.2 kg of fish a week, and bake or grill the fish -- don't fry it -- to keep it healthy.

Olive Oil: Olive oil is a plant-based fat, so it's a better choice when trying to lower "bad" cholesterol than animal fats. It's great with red wine vinegar, a minced garlic clove, and a little ground pepper for a salad dressing. Or try braising vegetables like carrots or leeks: just drizzle 3 tablespoons of oil over vegetables in a snug baking dish, scatter some herbs, cover with foil, and put in a 375-degree oven for about 45 minutes.
Soy milk magic: soy milk is high in protein, and 25 grams a day can reduce cholesterol by 5 percent. Top off your cereal with soy milk, or use tofu instead of meat in stir-fries.

Beans Bounties: Black or kidney beans and lentils are rich in soluble fibre, which binds to cholesterol and moves it out of the body. Recent studies show 4.5 kg of beans a day can reduce LDL levels by 5 percent. Beans are versatile, and the possibilities are endless.

Be Fruitful: Pears and apples have a lot of pectins, a fibre that can lower cholesterol. Citrus fruits too, like oranges, lemons and berries.

Veritable Veggies: Most vegetables are high in fibre and low in calories. Eggplant and okra contain high amounts of soluble fibre. Eggplants are also high in antioxidants. But any vegetable is rich in fibre and nutrients.

Fortified Foods: Natural chemicals called sterols, from plant foods, help your body absorb less cholesterol. Foods like yogurt, milk, orange juice, are now fortified with plant sterols, which contribute to reducing cholesterol levels by up to 15%.

Others include cereals, bread and soy milk. Just check the label to make sure you're not getting too many calories.

Balanced Diet: The body requires 13 essential vitamins on a regular basis just to function normally.
It is important that we look out for all the essentials we try to prepare or take a meal.

Fruit – Focus on whole fruits rather than juices for more fibre and vitamins and aim for 1½ to 2 servings or more each day. Break the apple and banana rut and go for colour-rich pickings like berries or melons.

Veggies – colour is your credo in this category. Choose antioxidant-rich dark, leafy greens, such as kale, spinach, and broccoli as well as orange and yellow vegetables, such as carrots, squash, and yams. Try for 2 to 2½ cups of veggies every day.

Calcium – Maintaining bone health as you age depends on adequate calcium intake to prevent osteoporosis and bone fractures. Older adults need 1,200 mg of calcium a day through servings of milk, yogurt, or cheese. Non-dairy sources include tofu, broccoli, almonds, and kale.

Grains – Be smart with your carbs and choose whole grains over processed white flour for more nutrients and more fibre. If you're not sure, look for pasta, loaves of bread, and cereals that list "whole" in the ingredient list. Older adults need 6-7 kg of grains each day (0.03kg is about 1 slice of whole grain bread).

Protein – Adults over 50 without kidney disease or diabetes need about 1 to 1.5 grams per kilogram of bodyweight. This translates to 68 to 102g of high-quality protein per day for a person weighing 0.5 g of protein per kg of body weight is close enough. Try to divide your protein intake equally among meals. It's important to vary your sources of protein instead of relying on red meat, including more fish, beans, peas, eggs, nuts, seeds, and low-fat milk and cheese in your diet.

Tips for Creating a Balanced Diet

It doesn't have to be difficult to swap a tired eating regimen for a tasty, well-balanced eating plan.

Avoid skipping meals – This causes metabolism to slow down, leading to sluggishness and poorer choices later in the day.

Breakfast – Select high-fibre bread and cereals, colourful fruit, and protein for a day's worth of energy. Try yogurt with muesli and berries, a veggie-packed omelette, peanut butter on whole grain toast with a citrus salad, or old-fashioned oatmeal made with dried cherries, walnuts, and honey.

Lunch – Keep your body fuelled for the afternoon with a variety of whole-grain bread, lean protein, and fibre. Try a veggie stew with whole-wheat noodles, or a quinoa salad with roasted peppers and mozzarella cheese.

Dinner – End the day on a wholesome note. Try warm salads of roasted veggies and a side of crusty brown bread and cheese, grilled salmon with spicy salsa, or whole-wheat pasta with asparagus and shrimp. Opt for sweet potatoes instead of white potatoes and grilled meat instead of fried.

Snacks – It's okay, even recommended, to snack. But make it count by choosing high-fibre snacks to tide you healthfully over to your next meal. Choose almonds and raisins instead of chips, fruit instead of sweets. Other smart snacks include yogurt, cottage cheese, apples and peanut butter, and veggies.

Chapter Seven

Eating Towards Productivity

Productivity is never an accident. It is always a result of a commitment to excellence, intelligent planning and focused effort.
- Paul I Meyer

Productivity is defined as a measure of the efficiency of a machine, person, system or tool.

However, our focus here is on how eating can affect your productivity. This time around, you are the tool or the machine.

When we think about the factors that contribute to workplace performance, we rarely give much consideration to food. For those of us battling to stay on top of emails, meetings, and deadlines, food is simply fuel. The foods we eat, affect us more than we realize.

Here's a brief rundown of why this happens. Our body converts everything we eat into glucose, which provides the energy our brains need to stay alert. When we're running low on glucose, we have a tough time staying focused and our attention drifts. This explains why it's hard to concentrate on an empty stomach.

Not all foods are processed by our bodies at the same rate. Some foods, like pasta, bread, cereal and soda, release their glucose quickly, leading to a burst of energy followed by a slump.

High-fat meals provide more sustained energy but require our digestive system to work harder, reducing oxygen levels in the brain.

Most of us know this, but because we are at our lowest thinking level when hungry, we don't make smart decisions. But again we need to make decisions and strategic ones at that if we are to be highly productive.

Here are some basic tips as to help you plan your lunch.

Make your eating decisions BEFORE **you get hungry**

It is pertinent and paramount at that. The reason being that you would be able to plan where you are going and what you want to eat. If you're going out to lunch, choose where you're eating in the morning, not at 12:30 PM. If you're ordering in, decide what you're having after a mid-morning snack. Studies show we're a lot better at resisting salt, calories, and fat in the future than we are in the present.

Don't wait till you are terribly hungry before eating.

This means that you should take healthy snacks before the main meal. Smaller, more frequent meals maintain your glucose at a more consistent level than relying on a midday feast.

Make healthy snacking easier to achieve than unhealthy snacking.

You could practice this by buying fruits which make snacking easy and healthy. Almonds are around and affordable, so you can get some and place them where your eyes can easily see them.

Research indicates that eating fruits and vegetables throughout the day isn't just good for the body also beneficial for the mind.

One of the fascinating things about eating is how various ingredients enter your brain through your blood stream. Whichever elements make it through to power your brain will help you to either focus or lose focus.

"The brain works best with about 25 grams of glucose circulating in the blood stream — about the amount found in a banana."
                                        -Leigh Gibson

It would interest you to know that you are in full control of how glucose gets into your blood stream. Certain foods release glucose quickly while others do so more slowly, yet sustainably

I will explain using two foods, donuts and oats.

After eating the donut, we will release glucose into our blood very quickly. You will have about 20 minutes of alertness. Then your glucose level will drop rapidly, leaving you unfocused and easy to distract. It's like putting the foot down on the pedal until you've used all your fuel.

The oats, on the other hand, will release their sugar as glucose much slower. This means we will have a steady glucose level, better focus and attention levels. Another important factor is your Leptin levels. Leptin will signal to your brain how full you are. If you now guess that a donut won't signal your brain to be full for a long time, while oats will, you're very right. We measure glycaemic index here (explains food's effect on a person's glucose level).

3 Most important aspects of getting the most out of eating food

Reorganize the positioning of food stored in your cupboard: One of the most interesting aspects of eating is that we are extremely likely to eat what is in close sight. You are more liable to eat the first thing you see in your cupboard than the fifth thing you see. Make sure you organize your food in a way that brain powering foods get more exposure. It's an incredible trick to start eating better food that will give you more daily alertness.

Learn to start with small portions: The brain needs very accurately portioned amounts of food. Too much will give you a spike that rapidly declines. Too little won't bring your brain up to speed. An excellent way to go about it, I've found, is to make your 3 daily meals a bit smaller (potentially by making the plates smaller). And then add 2 very specific, healthy snacks in between meals to keep your brain working at full speed. This way you don't have to change your core habits too much, yet can still fuel up your brain more efficiently.

Some foods are more brain powering than others, and those foods are to be consumed properly. Find such foods for example, nuts, seeds, chocolate.

Chapter Eight

Eating Right for Your Blood Type

I was reminded that my blood type is Be Positive
- Toluse Francis

Blood Type A

People with this type best show the powerful interconnections between mind and body. The Blood Type Diet's proactive mix of lifestyle strategies, hormonal equalizers, gentle exercise and specialized dietary guidelines, will maximize your overall health; decrease your inherent risk factors for cancer, diabetes and cardiovascular disease. The result: high performance, mental clarity, greater vitality and increased longevity.

Type A's have a naturally high level of the stress hormone cortisol and produce more in response to stressful situations. Cortisol is released in 24-hour patterns, typically in the early morning between six and eight with a gradual decrease during the day. Due to the naturally elevated cortisol in type As, additional stress often manifests in several ways; disrupted sleep patterns, daytime brain clout, increased blood viscosity (thickening), and promotes muscle loss and fat gain. In extreme cases in Type As, stress can manifest in more serious ways, causing obsessive-compulsive disorder, insulin resistance and hypothyroidism. To help balance cortisol levels, it is recommended that you limit sugar, caffeine and alcohol. Don't skip meals, especially breakfast; eating smaller, more frequent meals will also help to stabilize blood sugar levels. He also points out that the following factors are known to increase cortisol levels and increase mental exhaustion for Type A's - be aware and limit your exposure when possible to

- Crowds of people
- Loud noise
- Negative emotions
- Smoking
- Strong smells or perfumes
- Overwork
- Violent TV and movies
- Lack of sleep
- Extreme weather conditions (hot or cold)

In addition to exercise, stress management and eating the right foods, here are some key lifestyle strategies for Type A individuals.

- Cultivate creativity and expression in your life
- Establish a consistent daily schedule

- Go to bed no latest early and sleep for eight hours or more
- Take at least two breaks during the work day. Stretch, take a walk, do deep breathing exercises or meditate.
- Be righteous with eating
- Eat more protein at the start of the day
- Eat when relaxed
- Eat smaller, more frequent meals.
- Plan regular screening for heart disease and cancer prevention.
- Always chew food thoroughly to enhance digestion
- A meat-free diet based on fruits and vegetables, beans and legumes, and whole grains -- ideally, organic and fresh. People with type A blood have a sensitive immune system.

Type B Diet

Certain foods help weight gain stimulants for these categories. They are corn, wheat, lentils, tomatoes, peanuts and sesame seeds. Each of these foods affects the efficiency of your metabolic process, resulting in fatigue, fluid retention, and hypoglycaemia - a severe drop in blood sugar after eating a meal. When you eliminate these foods and begin eating a diet that is right for your type, your blood sugar levels should remain normal after meals.

Another very common food that Type Bs should avoid is chicken. Chicken contains a Blood Type B agglutinating lectin in its muscle tissue. Although chicken is a lean meat, the issue is the power of an agglutinating lectin attacking your bloodstream and the potential for it to lead to strokes and immune disorders.

It is suggested that you wean yourself away from chicken and replace them with highly beneficial foods such as goat, lamb, mutton, rabbit and venison. Other foods that encourage weight loss are green vegetables, eggs, beneficial meats, and low-fat dairy. These doesn't, however, rule out eating of vegetables totally but encouraged to have them in little quantity.

When the toxic foods are avoided and replaced with beneficial foods, Blood Type Bs are very successful in controlling their weight.

Live Healthy…

• Visualization is a powerful technique for Type Bs. If you can visualize it, you can achieve it

• Spend at least twenty minutes a day involved in some creative task that requires your complete attention

• Go to bed early and sleep for eight hours or more. It is essential for B's to maintain their circadian rhythm

• Use meditation to relax during breaks

• As they age, Type Bs have a tendency to suffer memory loss and have decreased mental activity. Stay sharp by doing tasks that require concentration, such as crossword puzzles or learn a new skill or language. Eating meals that enhance memory would be needful.

Type O blood

• Develop clear plans for goals and tasks – annual, monthly, weekly, daily to avoid impulsivity.

• Make lifestyle changes gradually, rather than trying to tackle everything at once.

• Eat all meals, even snacks, seated at a table.

- Chew slowly and put your fork down between bites of food. In essence, be calm while eating
- Avoid making big decisions or spending money when stressed.
- Do something physical when you feel anxious.
- When you crave a pleasure releasing-substance (alcohol, tobacco, sugar), do something physical.
- A high-protein diet heavy on lean meat, poultry, fish, and vegetables, and light on grains, beans, and dairy.

Type AB blood

Type AB reflects the mixed inheritance of their A and B genes. These set of people should avoid caffeine and alcohol, especially when you're in stressful situations.

Foods to focus on include tofu, seafood, dairy, and green vegetables. He says people with type AB blood tend to have low stomach acid and also avoid smoked or cured meats.

Chapter Nine

THE BALANCE

A balanced diet may be the best medicine- Anonymous

As an undergraduate at Bowen University, I realised that most females would order from a menu and have the following; rice, beans, meat, fish, egg and sometimes spaghetti I almost could tell what gender owned a particular meal once I see the plate.

So one day I decided to ask why they buy theirs that way and to my utmost shock, a lady said it's balanced diet. My mouth went agape.

I realised it was a matter of psychological satisfaction that was derived rather than eat a balanced diet after my interaction with some bevy of ladies.

I am very sure that many of us were only taught that we eat a balanced diet so we can have the three classes of food, especially at the secondary education level. But have you ever thought of what you could be gaining asides the specific right your balanced diet does to you?

Which do you think would give you energy the more a plate of rice, or a plate of beans?

I can hear you whisper 'rice of course.'

Hahaha...You are very wrong as they give you same quantity of energy. Did I say energy? Scratch those calories
So here is it...

Remember rice is carbohydrate while Beans is a protein.
Carbohydrates provide the same amount of energy in the form of calories as protein, with 4 calories per gram, but less than fat, with 9 calories per gram. Both starches and sugars provide you with energy.
Can you now see that you can feed on proteins and still not die?

But wait a second, the work of the calories in beans comes out when that of rice is depleted and onto the fats as the final source of help.
Hence, you won't feel weak until all the calories (glucose) in your body are depleted.
Your meals need present to us these three classes of food for energy sake, carbs, protein and fats.

Your meals should contain proteins and vitamins in the interests of bodybuilding. In this case, as explained above, the vitamins take over from the Protein in this function.

Your meals should contain vitamins and minerals for the sake of bone formation, healthy teeth and of course, body metabolic processes.

The key to healthy living and eating is striking a balance. It is essential that you strike a balance when thinking about that meal you want to eat.

Having an understanding that your carbohydrate cannot give you all nutrients needed by the body is the key to healthy living. This, by extension, suggests that you must have classes of food in the right proportion and at all times.

It is also not enough that you eat well but that you understand your lifestyle, your age, your blood group, just to mention few as they would help would help you have a well-planned diet.

It is not the quantity you that makes you healthy but the quality of the food. Eat purposefully and not aimlessly. Until you eat so as to stay healthy rather than to have your stomach filled, you may never eat well.

Conclusion

It is okay should you encounter some problems with eating. In that case, you can get a health coach who would take you through. A coach teaches and guides but an expert shows what he knows by telling you and leaving you to yourself. What you need when you hit the bricks is someone to showyou the way and walk with you.

In my experience as a coach, I have realised that many people know what to do but desire that someone shows them how to start and that such a person be available as they travel the journey.

Get one today if you have challenges with healthy eating.
Get in touch with me today as I am available to lead you through.

I run a coaching program known as The Eat Fit Program at the Eat Fit Academy

Join our Facebook Community where we share helpful tips and lessons.

To A Healthy Life!

Toluse Francis
2016

Contacts

www.tolufrancis.com
www.facebook.com/toluse.francis
www.twitter.com/Iamtolufrancis
www.linkedin.com/tolusefrancis
www.instagram.com/Iamtolufrancis
www.youtube.com/francistoluse
https://plus.google.com/u/1/+francistoluse
https://www.facebook.com/groups/eatfitacademy/